Thirty-One and a Half-Day Habit Shift

Simple Guide to Helping Ladies Over 40 Look and Feel Better... One Day at a Time

Matt Fruci

Thirty-One and a Half-Day Habit Shift

Independently published

Copyright © 2019, Matt Fruci

Published in the United States of America

190619-01410.3

ISBN: 9781697562392

Here's What's Inside...

Introduction

It's 2019, and here I am writing my second book just 2 years after my first one. I did think twice about this. After all, do you really need more information about weight loss, healthy eating and fitness? I would go as far as saying, if you just did what you already knew, you'd get the results you've always wanted.

After all, repetition is the mother of all skills. The more time you hear something, the more you take it in, the better. Sure, new information sometimes leads to new results but only if you execute. Even if you disagree with this, wouldn't it be fun to find out if it's true?

This is probably where the problem is; so-called 'experts' telling you to never eat carbs to cure Type 2 diabetes one minute and then blaming carbs the next. Oh, and don't forget that eating after 6pm makes you store more fat (I joke..), 5 weeks to sugar free, intimidating gyms with twenty year olds lifting heavy weights. It's frustrating.

You don't want to spend hours in an intimidating gym full of twenty-year-olds chucking weights around. You don't want to have to live off of detox shakes and skip meals with your loved ones. And it's confusing when one person says "eat what you want" and the other says "only eat green foods". I get it. You're busy and don't want to spend hours worrying about what you can and can't eat.

This brings me to this 31 and a half day habit transformation. From working with hundreds of ladies over 40 who struggle with emotional eating, self-sabotage and keeping going for long enough to see the results they want, my focus has shifted to breaking down this confusing nutrition and fitness world into small, simple DAILY habits so you can do the things you know you need to do. What's the best thing about this? Small habits have a compound effect. After all, where you are right now with your relationships, family, work, body and mind-set is a direct result of your daily habits over the past 30, 60, 90 and even 360 days and more.

As they say, if you just did what you already knew, you'd probably get the results you want. The point of this really is about repetition. The more you hear something, the more you take it in, and the more self-aware you become about what you are or are not doing. Most importantly, you can then question why you do the things that make you feel rubbish. The things you beat yourself up for doing. I mean, some people call it 'self-sabotage'.

The more I think about this, the more I believe that self-sabotage is not actually a thing. Hear me out on this. We don't just 'do something' for no reason. We do it because it's:

A) Convenient

B) Makes us feel good

Why wouldn't we do it? Examples:

- Eating takeaway – convenient and tasty

- Picking at biscuits – tastes good / takes us away from stress / boredom (albeit briefly)

- Convincing ourselves that we can't fit exercise in today...and that tomorrow will be easier. All these things make us feel better (albeit short term. I would even argue that they are more exhausting than actually doing the thing we know we need to do)

What can you do instead?

Well, I hope this book helps you with this by getting you to create a pattern interrupt aka something to do instead that is also:

A) Convenient

B) Makes us feel good

This has to be YOUR pattern interrupt. I cannot give you your pattern interrupt.

Examples include:

- Dancing
- Singing
- Sewing
- Taking a bath
- Reading
- Exercising (especially good if you feel "anger" or "anxiety")

So, what is the key part to this?

It is leverage. Leverage is something to pull you in the direction of understanding why you want to do it right now (or why you do not want to do it).

We go into this in more detail in Habit Shift 14. But be prepared to learn nothing new from me. You have the answers; I am just going to ask you the questions. I mean, new information sometimes does lead to new results, but only if you actually do it.

One of the things this book will help you overcome is looking for certainty before doing something. You know, the certainty that a diet will work, the certainty that it will help me lose one pound a week or two pounds a week, the certainty that it will be worth it. We want the certainty, but then the certainty actually stops us from doing, and actually finding out and getting clarity on what works and what doesn't work.

My point is that, the key really is in the doing. Even if you disagree with this, I always say, "Wouldn't it be fun to actually find out if it's true?" That the power comes from doing? It's probably where the problem is. You've got confusion, conflicting information, don't eat carbs, fruit is too high in sugar, avoid saturated fats, stop eating dairy, don't eat 'that' one minute, eat them the next, and never eat after 6pm because it makes us store fat. I could go on.

This is where this 31-and-a-half-day habit transformation comes in. After helping hundreds of ladies over 40 who struggle with emotional eating, self-sabotage, keeping going for long enough to see the results they want, I decided to simplify this process into 15 simple habits that you can fit into your lifestyle (even on your busiest day).

My focus has shifted from more information to actually breaking this down into small daily habits, so that you actually start doing the things that you probably know you already need to do. The best thing about this is that the small habits have a compound effect. Because where we are right now with our relationships, family, work, body, and mind-set is a direct result of our daily habits over the past 30-60-90 even 360 days.

You have to build momentum, build confidence in what you're doing so you can find out what doesn't work to give you the power to do more of what does work. You'll start to just do more, because you get confidence from doing it, even if you're getting 1% better each day. Because your mind can really only measure what we're going to lose, from doing something, but it can't really measure what we're going to gain from something.

My point is, when we often start a new habit, you often think of the reason why you can't do it. What you will lose from doing it. Yet, we don't consider what we'll gain from it. Take the simple habit of drinking water; a very simple habit. You know you should do it. Everyone does. So why do we not do it? Inconvenience? Yet, when you consider what the costs of not doing this habit are, your mind-set might just start to shift. Because by saying 'no' to drinking more water, you are essentially saying 'no' to more concentration, better digestion, more energy, better skin, less water retention, a stronger immune system, healthier organs, and I could go on. It can help fill you up, eat fewer calories, lose weight, and feel better. You could overcome the afternoon slump. Consider that you can't create new results while sticking with your old behaviours.

Again, that's pretty obvious, it's probably why you're reading the book, but then I want you to consider this: You cannot create new behaviours with your old beliefs. So then it's a case of questioning what your 'normal' is right now.

How you respond to situations, stress, whether you call foods 'bad', beat yourself up for not being perfect, calling yourself 'unfit' and 'fat', saying "I failed, I couldn't stick to this, I'll start Monday because it has to be perfect." You know this all or nothing mind-set.

This is where this comes in, to question your beliefs. Because ultimately, what you believe in, will impact how you feel, how you feel will impact what you do, and what you do will impact the results you get. Remember that it's you vs. you. The moment you compare yourself to others, you have just wasted energy that could've been spent on being the best version of you; the best version of you TODAY. What can you do today so that tomorrow you are better, even 1%. It could be as simple as walking for five minutes today and then walk five minutes and five seconds tomorrow. It's as simple as that; anyone can do it. Focus in on the fact that you could be one day away from seeing the results you want. Just imagine if you gave up because you didn't see the result on the scale, or how you look or how you feel, or someone didn't notice today. Yet, you were just one day away from someone noticing, the scale moving, getting the energy you want, and feeling better, fitter, and stronger? Imagine if you were one day away from changing your life?

This is why I put together these 15 habits, they'll be drip fed to you over the next 31 and a half days using this book, so you can start to build momentum, build your confidence, get 1% better each day, and remember that small habits have a compound effect. So you can just add them up, build momentum, transform your beliefs, how you feel, what you do, and essentially the results that you get. You can go from the all or nothing mind-set, to thinking something rather than nothing. Always think something rather than nothing.

My hope for you after reading this book is that you'll be inspired to actually put these habits into place and build momentum. You can think *something* rather than *all or nothing*. If you have one bad day, you can get back into the plan with a small daily win and do any of these habits, even on your busiest, most stressful day. Whenever you need a kickstart you can always go back to day one and just build again. Start over as many times as you want. As I said, after all, repetition is the mother of all skills. The more time you hear something, the more you take it in, the better. Sure, new information sometimes leads to new results but only if you execute.

Here's to your strongest days to come,

Matt

Is This Habit Worth It to Me?

Before I go revealing these habits to you, sit down and grab a coffee (that's a habit of mine, come to think of it) because I'm about to help you understand just how critical they are to your success in anything.

So, a habit is an automatic response developed via context-dependent repetition. In simple terms, we - as humans – have to make millions of decisions. It would be exhausting to even do the simple day-to-day things in life if we didn't have the ability to create habits. This means that we don't have to waste so much energy in making decisions. We become more efficient at doing 'stuff'. This can be said for so-called 'good' habits, such as going for a walk at lunchtime, and so-called 'bad' habits, such as raiding the cupboards for snacks whilst watching TV.

Now, the next question is often: "How do I break a bad habit?" The way I see it, is that you have to put your attention on what you will do instead and create new habits. So, rather than saying "don't snack", you focus on what you will do instead, be it going for a walk, doing some exercise, ringing a friend, reading, having a bath, or anything you find 'fun' or 'rewarding'. Like I said before, you have to add a habit in which is rewarding and convenient.

A powerful way to create new habits is to group it with things you already do. For example, most people know they need to drink more water for their skin, digestion, bloating, productivity, energy etc. Yet, people still forget. Something I do is to attach the new habit to an existing one. For example, I rarely leave the house in the morning without my coffee. So, every time I have a coffee, I have a glass of water. This almost puts this new habit on autopilot so even if I don't make a conscious effort to drink water at any other time of the day, I will still have around 3 glasses of water (as I usually have 3 cups of coffee a day).

Anyway, I named this chapter '*Is This Habit Worth It To Me?*' because I want you to consider this:

Habits are automatic. If you see a cue, your behaviour will follow. So, this is where we apply the one minute rule inside our Kickstart Programme, which relates to helping with comfort eating and snacking. This involves creating a pause before you act. So, next time you go to snack, give yourself the freedom to make the choice. Look at the food for one minute and ask yourself if you really want it. If you do want it, then enjoy it. The point here is the fact you give yourself the freedom of choice rather than bring a slave to your habits.

One last thing; do not beat yourself up just because it didn't work straight away. Habits are built over years and years. It will take time. But just like anything, the more you do something, the easier it will get. I always say to myself: "what would I tell my daughters if they said they were going to give up?"

As they say, the advice you give to others is often the advice you need to hear yourself.

How to Use
the Habit Shift

So, over the next pages, I will be setting you a habit to add in to your day. You will then see a checkbox for you to keep score of each day you do this habit. The book is designed so that you add in a new habit every two days. That being said, this is your journey. So, if you want to add in just one new habit a week, that's all good, too. The more important part of all of this is that you move in the right direction, no matter how fast or slow. As we say in our Kickstart Programme, just focus on getting 1% better today.

Habit Shift 1:
Eat Slowly

This is Task 1: Eat slowly – put your utensils down between bites to slow down your eating. This can combat mindless eating.

That's so simple...so why don't you do it?

Habit Shift 1: Eat Slowly

Track your progress below and score yourself over the next week by putting a 1 on the days you add the habit shift.

M	T	W	Th	F	Sat	Sun

Score: _____

Start this habit shift today. Keep score and see if you can add this habit shift each day.

What did you find when you did this habit?

_____

_____

_____

_____

Habit Shift 2:
Stop Eating at 80% Full

Did you know there's a difference between feeling full and having enough?

Ask yourself why you are eating.

- Is it hunger, or is it your environment?
- Boredom?
- Habit ("it's noon I must have lunch")?
- Because it's there?
- Tiredness?
- Stress?

Just acknowledging this and writing down the trigger will help you challenge your behaviour.

Remember, you only get results for DONE.

Habit Shift 2: Stop Eating at 80% Full

Track your progress below and score yourself over the next week by putting a 1 on the days you add the habit shift.

M	T	W	Th	F	Sat	Sun

Score: _____

Start this habit shift today. Keep score and see if you can add this habit shift each day.

What did you find when you did this habit?

_____

_____

_____

_____

Habit Shift 3:
Avoid Eating From a Package or Packet – Portion Your Food

We eat with our eyes. We tend to eat 92% of what we serve. So, if you've bought a big packet to 'save money' as the supermarkets have you believe, you are likely to eat more unless you portion it or buyer smaller pots. You can 'waist it' or 'waste it'.

Example: If I buy a big tub of Greek yoghurt or peanut butter, I'll eat more. Also, it's better value to buy meats in bulk from a butcher and get them to portion it up.

Habit Shift 3: Avoid Eating From a Package or Packet – ALWAYS Eat Pre-portioned Food

Track your progress below and score yourself over the next week by putting a 1 on the days you add the habit shift.

M	T	W	Th	F	Sat	Sun

Score: _____

Start this habit shift today. Keep score and see if you can add this habit shift each day.

What did you find when you did this habit?

_____

_____

_____

_____

Habit Shift 4:
Keep Your Counters Clear of All Foods Apart From Vegetables and Fruits

The more decisions you make, the less willpower you have and the more difficult it becomes to avoid the packet of biscuits or cereal set out on the side. You make 200 decisions every day about...food!

- What to eat

- When to eat

- How much to eat

- With a spoon, or in a bowl?

- What should they eat? Is this healthy?

Did you know that women who left cereal boxes out on the side tended to be 20 pounds heavier than their neighbours who didn't? Those who had sugary soft drinks out on the side tended to be 26 pounds heavier. Those who had a fruit bowl out were lighter by one to three pounds.

Habit Shift 4: Keep Your Counters Clear of All Foods Apart Form Vegetables and Fruits

Track your progress below and score yourself over the next week by putting a 1 on the days you add the habit shift.

M	T	W	Th	F	Sat	Sun

Score: _____

Start this habit shift today. Keep score and see if you can add this habit shift each day.

What did you find when you did this habit?

_____

_____

_____

_____

Habit Shift 5:
Eat Lean Protein with
Every Meal

*? lunch & supper
• not b'fast*

Lean protein has been shown to keep you full and give you a more toned look. Research has shown that when you eat protein with each meal, you subconsciously eat less. Could this be because protein is essential for your body and you have to get it from your diet? After all, it's important for your skin, hair, nails, digestion, muscles, and more. For example, protein might include Greek yoghurt, eggs, chicken, turkey, beef, pork, fish, soy, tofu, beans, and legumes.

How do you know if it's a lean meal?

<u>Key words when choosing your protein:</u>

* 'loin', 'roast', 'T-bone', 'tenderloin', 'skirt', 'sirloin', 'fish'

<u>Key words to look for in a meal:</u>

* Baked, broiled, boiled, fresh, grilled, marinated, poached, roasted, seasoned, steamed, vinaigrette

<u>Words to be wary of:</u>

* 'A La Crème', 'basted', 'bottomless', 'breaded', 'buttered', 'cheesy', 'carbonara', 'golden', 'crispy', 'platter', 'stuffed', 'smothered'

This is what a portion of protein looks:

Aim for - roughly - a palm-sized portion of protein. This will give you around 20g of protein at a meal (which has been shown to keep you full up and curb cravings)

Habit Shift 5: Eat Lean Protein with Every Meal

Track your progress below and score yourself over the next week by putting a 1 on the days you add the habit shift.

M	T	W	Th	F	Sat	Sun

Score: _____

Start this habit shift today. Keep score and see if you can add this habit shift each day.

What did you find when you did this habit?

_____

_____

_____

_____

Habit Shift 6:
Eat At Least 5 Servings of Colourful Vegetables and Types of Fruit

Vegetables and fruits are full of antioxidants, vitamins and minerals. All of these help with ageing, skin, hair, nails, as well as boosting your immune system. (Notice how I said vegetables and fruits and not fruits and vegetables?)

These vegetables and fruits also help to keep you full up and satisfied by giving your body the nutrients and energy it needs. Of course, there's more. The fibre found in vegetables and fruits can help fight against cancer, Type 2 Diabetes, and heart disease. You may also want to regulate your fibre intake should you have digestive issues.

Aim for a minimum of three portions of veggies and a maximum of two portions of fruit per day.

A portion is the amount you can cup in your hand, but feel free to go crazy on veggies (as long as your digestive system allows you to).

Can I challenge you to get 5 in today?

Habit Shift 6: Eat at Least 5 Servings of Colourful Vegetables and Types of Fruit

Track your progress below and score yourself over the next week by putting a 1 on the days you add the habit shift.

M	T	W	Th	F	Sat	Sun

Score: _____

Start this habit shift today. Keep score and see if you can add this habit shift each day.

What did you find when you did this habit?

_____

_____

_____

_____

Do need 3 × 6 (cc4/16)

Habit Shift 7:
Take a Fish Oil/Omega-3 Capsule Every Morning

Found in oily fish such as salmon, trout, mackerel and sardines, Omega-3s are associated with:

- A decreased risk of heart disease

- Increased ability to absorb and use protein so you can get that leaner look

- Increased concentration so you don't have to rely on caffeine to get through your day

- Healthier joints, so you hear fewer 'creaks'

- Improved gut health and a boosted immune system, so you spend less time with the sniffles and more time doing what you want to do!

The 'Fishing' Line:

- Eat oily fish at least two or three times per week (salmon, trout, mackerel, sardines)

- OR

- Consider supplementing with Omega-3 fish oil

Habit Shift 7: Take a Fish Oil/Omega-3 Capsule Every Morning

Track your progress below and score yourself over the next week by putting a 1 on the days you add the habit shift.

M	T	W	Th	F	Sat	Sun

Score: _____

Start this habit shift today. Keep score and see if you can add this habit shift each day.

What did you find when you did this habit?

_____

_____

_____

_____

Habit Shift 8:
Aim to Drink At Least 2 Litres of Water Per Day

Now, this is a starting point because the amount of fluid you will need depends on the weather, your exercise levels, and lifestyle.

These are some rules to go by:

- You're urinating clear by midday

- You're having three clear urinations a day; you're probably good to go!

Why bother? The following can be impacted by drinking plenty of water:

- Hunger

- Skin

- Energy

- Digestion

- Irritable Bowel Syndrome (IBS)
- Bloating
- Absorption
- How you feel

There's no time like the present; have a glass of water.

Habit Shift 8: Aim to Drink At Least 2 Litres of Water a Day

Track your progress below and score yourself over the next week by putting a 1 on the days you add the habit shift.

M	T	W	Th	F	Sat	Sun

Score: _____

Start this habit shift today. Keep score and see if you can add this habit shift each day.

What did you find when you did this habit?

_____

_____

_____

_____

Habit Shift 9:
Drink Only Calorie-Free Beverages

Liquid calories APART from protein shakes have been shown to trigger hunger. These hunger-triggering drinks include fizzy drinks and juices.

Simple swaps:

- Swap your latte for an Americano (milk is OK)

- Diet drinks instead of full sugar drinks

- Sugar-free squash instead of juice

Drink more water (herbal teas are fine, too). This is You vs You, remember, so no matter how small a change you make, don't forget that $1 > 0$:-)

Close the gap between where you are right now and where you want to be each day. That's the secret to losing weight and keeping it off, once and for all.

Habit Shift 9: Drink Only Calorie-Free Beverages

Track your progress below and score yourself over the next week by putting a 1 on the days you add the habit shift.

M	T	W	Th	F	Sat	Sun

Score: _____

Start this habit shift today. Keep score and see if you can add this habit shift each day.

What did you find when you did this habit?

_____

_____

_____

_____

Habit Shift 10:
Create Your Sleep Ritual

Altering your lifestyle habits, routines and behaviours does impact your sleep.

Stress >> escalated by tiredness >> binge and eat your emotions >> feel like a failure >> start again Monday.

This isn't your fault. It's sometimes a simple case of not prioritising the things that are important to you. This leads to you spending more time on the things that you need to do but won't give you the rewards you want the MOST.

For example, every evening, my daughter MUST have some food, her bath, and a little massage before going off to sleep. It's her ROUTINE.

These are ten things to consider when creating your new bedtime routine to improve your sleep, get more energy, and improve the way you handle food and burn fat.

1. **Be Regular:** Go to bed and get up at the same time (your body loves consistency).

2. **Stop working at the SAME time each day:** Have a power-down hour before bed (read, talk to your family...take your foot off the accelerator).

3. **Turn off the iPhone, iPad, and TV:** If that's how you 'relax', that's fine; just avoid too much light in the 30 minutes before bed. Try putting your TV on a timer, so it switches off...as you do.

4. **Read/meditate before bed**

5. **Exercise:** If this gives you energy, try to avoid it later in the day...but if it mellows you out, then do it later in the day!

6. **Get some light in the morning:** Go for a walk during the day or even at lunch.

7. **Protect your confidence:** Note down three things you did well that day, because where your attention goes, your energy goes. Remind yourself every day of what you did well. It could be you went to bed early so you feel more relaxed, planned your meals for tomorrow, took time for you, or went on a date with the other half. Maybe you exercised and practiced self-care, you practiced gratitude, and realised how 99% of stuff doesn't matter

In fact, try this:

Will you remember what you are worrying about in 48 Hours?

NO

Then it doesn't matter.

Will you remember what you are worrying about in one week?

NO

Then it doesn't matter.

Will you remember what you are worrying about in one month?

NO

Then it doesn't matter.

Will you remember what you are worrying about in one year?

NO

Then it doesn't matter.

Will you remember what you are worrying about on your deathbed?

NO

Then it doesn't matter.

To put things into perspective, 99% of the things you think matter, don't.

Save your energy for those times when things do matter and are life-changing.

For the rest of it, adapt and overcome to maintain your journey.

8. **Stay hydrated BUT:** Don't drink too close to bedtime; the rule is similar for eating as this can make you get up in the night;

9. **Try taking Magnesium Citrate for a weak bladder if you're up in the night weeing!**

10. **Avoid caffeine after 4 pm:** It can disrupt your sleep, leading to an inability to make better-informed, more intelligent decisions about the food you eat and weight gain.

So, there you have it.

Which one can you do today?

Habit Shift 10: Create Your Sleep Ritual

Track your progress below and score yourself over the next week by putting a 1 on the days you add the habit shift.

M	T	W	Th	F	Sat	Sun

Score: _____

Start this habit shift today. Keep score and see if you can add this habit shift each day.

What did you find when you did this habit?

_____

_____

_____

_____

Habit Shift 11:
Do Something That Makes You HAPPY Today (and I Mean Happy)

Why? Well, how do you feel when you have fun? Happy, right? When you're happy, you're not stressed. When you're not stressed, your mind is no longer full of the stuff that's stressing you out, and you're less likely to fall into this trap:

Stress >> escalated by tiredness >> binge and eat your emotions >> feel like a failure >> start again Monday.

So, today, I challenge you to do 30 minutes of something FUN for you. It could be anything. Watch your favourite TV programme, go for a walk, have a bath, ring a friend you haven't spoken to for a while. Anything!

Here's a task. Grab a pen and paper. Write down five things that make you feel happy. During the next time you feel down? Do one.

1.

2.

3.

4.

5.

These are some of my examples:

- Write a blog
- Date night with Mrs. Fruci
- Make my daughters laugh
- Exercise
- Drink a coffee and sit
- Watch/listen to comedy
- Deep breathing
- See family and friends
- Go to the beach

If I haven't done any of these, can I be happy?

Don't forget to put it in your diary. If you don't, you won't know where your time has gone, and you will always be time poor.

Habit Shift 11: Do Something That Makes You HAPPY Today (and I Mean Happy)

Track your progress below and score yourself over the next week by putting a 1 on the days you add the habit shift.

M	T	W	Th	F	Sat	Sun

Score: _____

Start this habit shift today. Keep score and see if you can add this habit shift each day.

What did you find when you did this habit?

_____

_____

_____

_____

Habit Shift 12:
Only Eat When You Have Sat Down

Eating when standing or on the go can mean you eat more than you think. Your body is stressed, and your hunger signals may not work so well as you are too occupied and not present at the moment. This can lead to mindless eating and that slow, gradual weight gain that we usually put down to 'getting older'.

Could it be that we're struggling to manage the increased stress and using food as comfort? So, from today on, you can only eat when you have sat down :-)

Habit Shift 12: Only Eat When You Have Sat Down

Track your progress below and score yourself over the next week by putting a 1 on the days you add the habit shift.

M	T	W	Th	F	Sat	Sun

Score: _____

Start this habit shift today. Keep score and see if you can add this habit shift each day.

What did you find when you did this habit?

_____

_____

_____

_____

Habit Shift 13:
Turn Off All Electricals
Whilst You Eat

Enjoy and savour every mouthful. Notice the texture and taste. Find out where the food came from. Be grateful.

Habit Shift 13: Turn Off All Electricals Whilst You Eat

Track your progress below and score yourself over the next week by putting a 1 on the days you add the habit shift.

M	T	W	Th	F	Sat	Sun

Score: _____

Start this habit shift today. Keep score and see if you can add this habit shift each day.

What did you find when you did this habit?

_____

_____

_____

_____

Habit Shift14: Crush Self-Sabotage

Grab a pen and answer these questions and keep them somewhere to remind yourself every... single...day:

- What is the behaviour that is stopping you from closing the gap between where you are now and where you want to be?

- What are the benefits of doing that behaviour? (Example: If the behaviour is eating chocolate, maybe (a) you get some comfort, (b) you have finished work, or (c) it's quick and easy.)

- What are the costs of this behaviour? (Examples: your integrity, feeling rubbish about yourself, not getting results)

- Are you going around in circles? (What has this cost you in the past?)

- What might happen if you don't get a handle on this? Health? Family time? Everyday tasks? Happiness?

This is where you get the leverage to pull you in the right direction.

How will you create a pattern interrupt to change your behaviour? An example would be that you have a bath or go for a walk after dinner to get out of the kitchen when you would normally snack.

Habit Shift 14: Crush Self-Sabotage

Track your progress below and score yourself over the next week by putting a 1 on the days you add the habit shift.

M	T	W	Th	F	Sat	Sun

Score: _____

Start this habit shift today. Keep score and see if you can add this habit shift each day.

What did you find when you did this habit?

_____

_____

_____

_____

Habit Shift 15:
Put Yourself First
You're No Good to Anyone When You're Tired, Stressed Out, and Lacking Patience

HALF-DAY BONUS

Answer these questions:

What is today's date?

_____

What is the date in 30 days?

_____

What do you want to have happened by this date?

sensible diet

Why is this important?

be healthier

What happens if you don't do it?

cross i no will power. poss. less t—

What are you willing to do to get there?

try slightly diff food - spend more money

Your 30-Day Habit Shift is now done and dusted!

But - as a little bonus for you - I've decided to put all of the 15 habits into one Cheat Sheet so you can keep score on how you're doing.

It's a big part of what we do in our Kickstart Programme; if you're not assessing, you're guessing. So, go to **www.FruciFit.com/HabitChecklist** to get it and score yourself each week out of 105 (1 point for each day of the week you DO your 15 habits)

How did you do?

RECAP:

1. Eat slowly
2. Stop at 80% full
3. Avoid eating from a packet or package
4. Keep your counters clear of all food apart from veggies and fruit
5. Eat lean proteins with every meal
6. Eat at least five portions of veggies or fruits
7. Take a fish oil or Omega-3 each morning
8. Drink at least 2 litres of water per day
9. Drink only calorie-free beverages
10. Create your sleep ritual
11. Do something fun
12. Only eat when you have sat down
13. Turn off all electricals whilst you eat
14. Crush self-sabotage and comfort eating
15. Put yourself first

(**Day 31.5**) Get clarity on your priorities

What Next

We've all been on a diet before and lost weight. The most challenging part is keeping it off so we can keep the results and feel better about the way we look and feel for good. The secret to this? Finding a way of eating that fits your lifestyle (and doesn't leave you feeling guilty for eating your favourite foods or beating yourself up for not being 'perfect') and allows you to fit exercise into your lifestyle without it being a time-consuming chore.

Many ladies think they're too unfit to start, have to give up their favourite foods for good, and spend hours exercising to lose weight, fit into the clothes they want to wear and get fit. I hope this book inspires you to focus on being 1% better every day so you can finally ditch the 'all or nothing' diet mind-set and focus on the fact that 'something is better than nothing'. In other words, 'half-assed is better than no assed'.

That's where our 4-Week Kickstart Programme comes in for ladies over 40 who want to overcome 'self-sabotage', kickstart their motivation and feel better about the way they look & feel. Our nutrition and fitness system is specifically designed for ladies 40+ who struggle to do the things they know they need to do.

If you'd like me to help you, go to **www.FruciFit**.com and click the **APPLY NOW** button and I'll send over the details for you.

Step 1: Go to **www.FruciFit.com** and click the **APPLY NOW** button.

Step 2: I'll get you started with your kickstart coaching session, where together, we'll go through your personalised plan & get you set up on our "*3F It*" *Accountability & Nutrition* system so you don't have to rely on willpower and can kickstart your health and fitness habits TODAY.

Step 3: You will receive ongoing support and accountability and be empowered to take control of your habits so you can build a diet and fitness plan to last. We'll closely monitor how you respond and adapt your plan based on your progress so you can DO IT even on your busiest, most stressful week.

"What if you were just one day away from getting the results you want... but you gave up?
- Matt Fruci

Made in the USA
Lexington, KY
05 November 2019

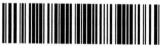